UNDERSTANDING BRAIN DISEASE

UNDERSTANDING BRAIN DISEASE

DR. JOSEPH B. MARTIN

DEAN, HARVARD MEDICAL SCHOOL

Introduction by Dr. Alastair M. Buchan
University of Oxford

The Inaugural
Margarete Wuensche Memorial Lecture

BAYEUX

UNDERSTANDING BRAIN DISEASE
© 2005 by Bayeux Arts, Inc.
119 Stratton Crescent SW,
Calgary, Canada T3H 1T7
www.bayeux.com

Library and Archives Canada Cataloguing in Publication
Martin, Joseph B., 1938-
      Understanding brain disease / Joseph B. Martin.
      ISBN 1-896209-65-3
  1. Brain--Diseases. I. Bayeux Arts (Firm) II. Title.
RC386.M37 2005   616.8   C2005-901512-8

First Printing: September 2005
Printed in Canada at Friesens

Books published by Bayeux Arts are available at special quantity discounts to use as premiums and sales promotions, or for use in corporate training programs. For more information, please write to Special Sales, Bayeux Arts, Inc., 119 Stratton Crescent SW, Calgary, Canada T3H 1T7.

The ongoing publishing activities of Bayeux Arts, under its "Bayeux" and "Gondolier" imprints, are supported by the Canada Council for the Arts, the Alberta Foundation for the Arts, and the Government of Canada through the Book Publishing Industry Development Program.

Dedicated to the memory of
Margarete Wuensche

Contents

Introduction

It gives me great pleasure to write this introduction for the first lecture given by Dr. Joe Martin on Neurodegenerative Brain Disorders.

These lectures are in memory of Margarete Wuensche.

Margarete Wuensche had a wonderful life and a very wonderful family. She lived extremely well and had a very short illness as a result of a stroke. Her death was unexpected as is so often the case with stroke. Mercifully, she was saved from a period of disability and she suffered little. Indeed, it was her family who suffered a great deal, but they too were spared the burden of caring for a disabled Margarete and the pain of seeing a loved one forever changed by neurological disease.

Richard Doll, who discovered the link between tobacco and cancer, has often remarked that one would want to die as young as possible but as old as possible. Indeed, Margarete was as young as possible but, sadly, died before her time.

Shortly after her death, I met with Caroline and Rolf, Margarete's daughter and husband, and we decided to create a series of lectures in connection with the Faculty of Medicine at the University of Calgary, Canada, to bring interesting lecturers to the Faculty with as wide a range of interests as possible.

These lectures are designed, in part, to bring new information about neurological disease to the public and, importantly, to bring literature, the arts, and other sciences back to neuroscience.

I was delighted to be able to recruit Joe Martin to give the first of the Wuensche Lectures. Joe is currently Dean of Medicine at Harvard Medical School and is a clinician and a neuroscientist. His formative years were spent not far from Calgary in Duchess, Alberta, and he graduated to the University of Alberta where he took his medical degree before specializing in neurosciences at McGill in Montreal.

Following a period of training, he spent time at Harvard and ultimately became a Chief of Neurology back at McGill before becoming the Head of Neurology at the Harvard Medical School. In a few short years, he then became the Dean of Medicine at the University of California, San Francisco and ascended to Olympian heights becoming the Chancellor of UCSF living on the top of Mt.

Parnassus overlooking San Francisco and the Bay Area.

From there, Joe has become the Dean of Harvard Medical School, one of medicine's glittering prizes along with such posts as Osler's Chair, the Regius Professorship at Oxford, or the Headship of the NIH.

We were delighted to welcome Joe back to his home in Alberta to give the first lecture, "Proteins, Plaques, and Prions". The lecture was delivered in Calgary on March 12, 2004, and is now being published by Bayeux Arts, a Calgary-based publisher, as *Understanding Brain Disease*.

We look forward to many subsequent lectures in Margarete's honor, and in particular, the lecture for 2005 which will be given by Dr. Oliver Sacks, the noted author and neurologist from New York.

Alastair Buchan,
Professor of Clinical Geratology,
University of Oxford,
England.

1 April 2005

Neurodegenerative Brain Disorders

We live in exciting times. They present enormous opportunities for understanding how the brain works and how to treat the illnesses that affect it, particularly as we grow older and become more familiar with the impact of aging on brain function. The things you read about in the Tuesday *New York Times* or in the *Scientific American* are the things which cross our paths as scientists as we think about the future. It was in that context that I was thinking about some of the current issues of our time:

- Stem cells
- Neurodegeneration
- Mad cows
- Infectious Proteins-Prions
- Brain Plasticity
- Animal Models of Disease

In what follows, I will cover many of these one way or

another. I will not profess to deal with them exhaustively, but I will touch on each of them.

I offer three points which I suggest we should have in mind as we move forward. Of course, we are all interested in treatments that will offer new hope. Getting to those treatments and proving them to be successful will occur only with carefully constructed clinical trials. I will be the first to say that we need to be careful not to over-hype the possibilities. For example, fifteen years ago gene therapy was going to fix everything. Yet, other than in some of the immune pathologies of childhood, gene therapy has not proved to be successful in a distinctive case of any significance. We need to be careful that we are honest and say what is really possible.

To begin, let me offer a definition of neurodegenerative diseases. These occur usually out of the blue as sporadic illnesses. They may be inherited too, and we will look at some of those in a moment. They are progressive, and usually come on in adults. They generally affect both sides of the brain so that their presentations are bilateral. Occasionally at the onset, like in Parkinson's disease, they may occur more on one side than the other. The symptoms of these diseases are caused by the death of neurons in the brain.

Disease	Number of U.S. Patients	Remarks
Lou Gehrig's Disease (ALS)	15,000	Motor neuron disease
Prion disease	~ 400	Number may rise in UK - about 150 cases from cattle
Alzheimer's	4,000,000	Incidence is 1 in 3 by age 85
Parkinson's	500,000	L-dopa does not stop the disease
Frontotemporal dementia (FTD)	~ 30,000	Includes Pick's disease
Huntington's	10,000	Triplet repeat disorder

Table 1

The most common of these diseases are listed on Table 1, and I will ask you to bear with me as we go through some of the names that you will all recognize, just to give you some sense of the prevalence of them in the United States. I am very aware that the population of Canada is about 10% of that of the U.S., so you can make those numbers. These illnesses will occur in both Canada and the U.S. in about equal numbers.

Let me start with Lou Gehrig's disease, an amyotrophic lateral sclerosis that struck the famous Yankee baseball player after whom the disease is named. It is a relatively rare disease that affects about 15,000 patients in the U.S. It is caused by the death of neurons that move our muscles, whether they are muscles of the arms or legs or the muscles of the swallowing and facial apparatus.

Prion disease is the one we all have learned about since the "mad cow" epidemic that began in England in the early '90s. I would remind you that the occurrence of Creutzfeldt-Jakob disease, which is the sporadic form of this disorder, is very rare; about one case per million people per year. Despite all the cows that were killed in the United Kingdom, and I will come back to that later, there were only about 150 proven instances of the variant form of Bovine Spongiform

4

Encephalopathy (BSE) in Europe.

The most common neurodegenerative disease is Alzheimer's disease. There are an estimated 4 million patients in the U.S. Among people of age over 85, its incidence is 1 in 3, and in some studies it has been found to be as much as 1 in 2.

Parkinson's disease is a relatively common disease. The important point about Parkinson's disease is despite its successful treatment with L-Dopa, its progression does not, in fact, stop.

Frontotemporal dementia is a condition that we have learned about only in the last 15 years. It used to be referred to in some cases as Pick's Disease.

Huntington's disease is almost always inherited. It is a relatively common disorder that is caused by a very specific genetic mutation called Triplet repeat disorder.

I will focus on some of these diseases, beginning with Alzheimer's. In 1906, and later in 1907, Alois Alzheimer, working in Heidelberg and Munich, described a woman of age 51 years who died with a rapidly progressive loss of memory, intellect, and cognitive function. He looked at the brain — he was a neuropathologist and also a psychiatrist — and found the changes that I will describe in a moment. During the course of the 20th century, the first carefully observed biochemical abnormality was acetylcholine deficiency in the brains of Alzheimer's patients. This remains the principal basis for treatment, which seeks to improve memory, even today. The abnormality was shown in the 1980s to be due to loss of nerve cells, specifically in the nucleus basalis, that make acetylcholine and send it to the brain. In 1984, with the identification of the structure of the protein that occurs in the center of the senile plaque, or the neuritic plaque, we began a period now known as the cell biology and molecular genetics era.

In 1907, Alzheimer described three things that led to his now-famous report, an extraordinary one viewed in retrospect. He described neurofibrillary tangles in nerve cells of the brain, he described senile or neuritic plaques, and then a less well-understood change called granulovacuolar degeneration in cells of the hippocampus, which is where memory is stored. Later in 1938, Scholz, also working in Germany, became the first to show that the amyloid changes in the brain could also occur in blood vessels and some form of that condition could lead to brain hemorrhages. Then, in the

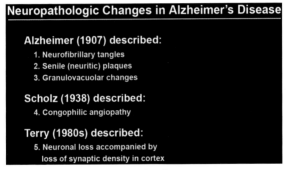

Neuropathologic Changes in Alzheimer's Disease

Alzheimer (1907) described:
1. Neurofibrillary tangles
2. Senile (neuritic) plaques
3. Granulovacuolar changes

Scholz (1938) described:
4. Congophilic angiopathy

Terry (1980s) described:
5. Neuronal loss accompanied by loss of synaptic density in cortex

Table 2

1980s, Terry and his colleagues began to demonstrate that the real cause of memory loss in Alzheimer's was due to the loss of the synaptic connections between nerve cells, which help us do everything that the brain accomplishes for us.

The neuropathology that Alzheimer described

consisted of neuronal neurofibrillary tangles which were seen under the electron microscope as paired helical filaments and was shown, subsequently, to be due to a protein which was excessively phosphorylated. The senile plaques with an amyloid core and, very importantly, the zone of inflammation around the senile plaque indicate that the toxicity of the amyloid is causing brain damage in the form of inflammation.

Here we have, in a silver stain, a typical neurofibrillary tangle — seen at the center of Figure 1 as two elongated, black staining clumps of the protein amyloid — in the cytoplasm of a cell. This cell is on its way to dying and surrounding it, in parts of the brain, are more of these clumps, which look like scars or deposits in the brain that consist of amyloid deposits, and the nerve fibers that come into there show degeneration in the form of these silver staining fibers.

If one does an amyloid stain (Figure 2), which is a special way to demonstrate the protein, one will find in the center of the senile plaque a dense deposit of the

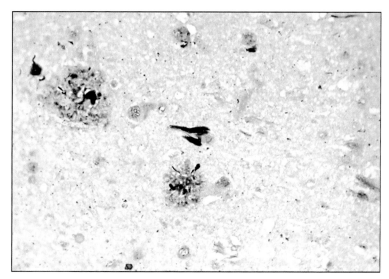

Figure 1

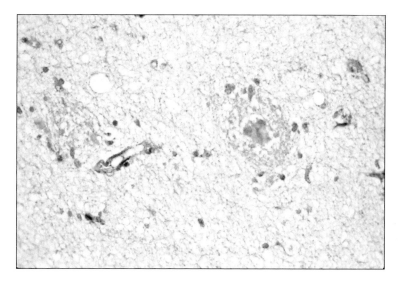

Figure 2

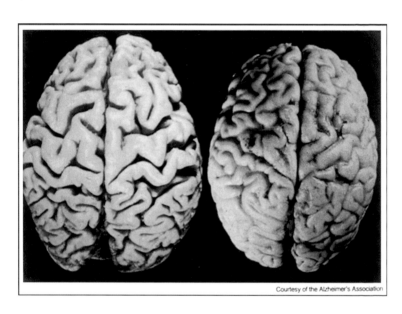

Figure 3

protein β-amyloid and that protein is well known as part of the fundamental understanding of Alzheimer's.

Let us attempt to describe how that protein does the damage that it appears to do. Notice here also that amyloid is deposited in the tiny blood vessels within the brain and occasionally those can rupture and cause a hemorrhage into the brain. The result of these two changes as they progress over the years is cortical atrophy or loss of the formations of the brain that we call gyri. On the right hand side of Figure 3 is a normal brain that has plump gyri and the spaces between those, the sulci, are very narrow and tight. In the case of Alzheimer's, on the left, the marked loss of the fullness of the gyri and the gaps that appear between them are associated with the loss of nervous tissue in the cerebral cortex. It is particularly prominent in the hippocampus, the region of the temporal lobe that we associate with memory formation.

Single Point Mutation

What we need now is some basic information on molecular genetics to help us understand the progress that has been made. Let us remind ourselves that everything we know about the way we are made and the way we function comes from the three billion base pairs of DNA which are found in each one of our cells. Let's take a look at Figure 4. The top part shows how the bases are paired to form these interesting connections between the two strands of DNA. The code for making the proteins that make the structure to function in our cells is also shown in the figure. The messenger RNA picks up the code from three of these base pairs and takes that genetic code of three to form each of the 20 amino acids we have. Proteins, which form the structure for everything that we currently know about ourselves, are simply chains of amino acids.

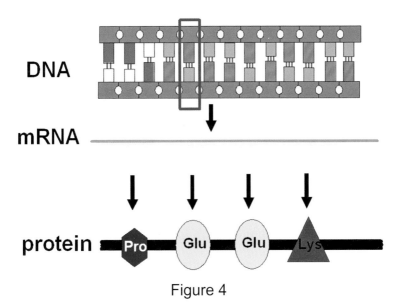

DNA

mRNA

protein   Pro   Glu   Glu   Lys

Figure 4

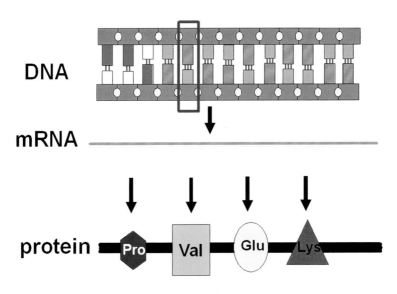

DNA

mRNA

protein   Pro   Val   Glu   Lys

Figure 5

If we take a single base pair, outlined in blue in the figure, and cause a mutation in it so that there is a missed signature or an error in the alphabet of that DNA, then we can get a change in one single amino acid (Figure 5). That single change is called a point mutation, a single mutation that can cause some of the most remarkable diseases known to humans.

I present an example. Probably the first disease to be identified in humans as a point mutation was

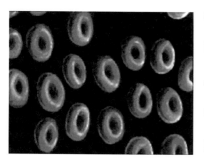

sickle-cell anemia, which is very common in African Americans. Figures 6 and 7 show how a single point mutation in the gene for hemoglobin produces

Figure 6: Normal cells

a dramatic structural change in the cells that look not perfectly formed like donuts, but are in fact sickle in a very abnormal way.

Now we know how dramatic a structural change a single point mutation can cause. Let me hasten to add that despite the fact that this mutation was demonstrated way back in 1975 and we now know the molecular basis of sickle-cell anemia, we

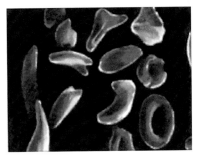

Figure 7: Sickle cells

still do not have a molecular treatment for the disease. This is a salutary reminder of how complex molecular structures are in genetic diseases. We should not imagine that we can just quickly fix them.

About Alzheimer's

Alzheimer's presents an example of one disease we are still working on. Table 3 looks at the progress in the understanding of Alzheimer's disease over the last century. The details are not important at this point. Simply, it tells us how science unfolds, how science evolves, and how discovery occurs with the new things that come along to enable one to do deeper penetrations into the mysteries of life and disease. Let's look at the chart and start with Alzheimer reporting the first case in 1906-07. The next big event happened in 1975, that of observing acetylcholine deficiency in patients afflicted with the disease. Amyloid peptide was purified by Glenner and Wong in 1984, and the first linkage was found on chromosome 21 in cases of familial Alzheimer's disease (FAD), which occurs in less than 10% of all cases. The gene for the amyloid protein was actually identified and cloned in 1987.

Progress in Alzheimer's Disease Research

1906: Alois Alzheimer reports first case

.

.

.

1975: ACh deficiency found in AD patients

1984: Amyloid peptide purified (Glenner & Wong)

1987: a) 1st FAD linkage found on chromosome 21

     b) APP gene cloned

1991: APP mutations found in FAD

1992: APOE identified as risk factor

1993: Presenilin 1 & 2 mutations discovered

1995: Transgenic mouse created with amyloid plaques

1998: Mutations found in tau

1999: a) Plaques clear after A-beta immunization

     b) Tangles seen in transgenic mice

     c) Secretases identified

2000: New clinical trials begin

Table 3

Then, over the course of the next three or four years, several specific genes that caused early onset of familial Alzheimer's were identified. Amyloid peptide itself had mutations in two genes — PS 1 and PS 2 — and association with apolipoprotein E, a certain form of blood protein.

Transgenic mice were first made in 1995 which carried the genes for Alzheimer's. They developed the plaques which I have just talked about, and they have become important models for testing drugs that might benefit the condition. Mutations were found in the tau protein in the neurofibrillary tangles in 1998 and then we began to look at real treatment possibilities with the finding that $A\beta$ immunization (giving the vaccine for the $A\beta$ protein to animals) could actually clear the plaques out of the brain. Other discoveries too were made, for which I will offer more details.

The leading hypothesis about Alzheimer's disease is that widely dispersed deposition of $A\beta$ throughout the brain causes the cells to die. There are three points here that emphasize why that seems likely. Many different genetic causes lead to one pathologic end point — the deposition of Aβ in the brain — which will be demonstrated as we go on. Secondly, Aβ, particularly in its most immature form of fibrils, is very toxic to the brain; nerve cells die. There is a general good correlation between the deposition of this material in the brain and the dementia that patients exhibit clinically.

We will now have to digress a little into biochemistry because I think it is very important to understand how we link together the possible discoveries of treatments that might make a difference in a condition like this.

This peptide, Aβ, comes from a larger protein called the amyloid precursor protein (APP). In its normal situation it sits right in the cell membrane of nerve cells and it has a long piece of the protein that sticks out the side of the cell and a shorter piece that sticks inside the cell. The part in Aβ in which we are particularly interested is the red piece in the middle of this protein (Figure 8). In the normal circumstance, it is manufactured in the cell, as all proteins are, and moves to the cell membrane where it does its work and is destroyed by enzymes that take it away. The normal cleavage as we call it is associated with an enzyme called α-secretase (a protein chopping molecule). In Alzheimer's disease, the abnormal cleavage occurs when key enzymes called β-secretase and γ-secretase, chopper enzymes cutting our proteins, produce an excessive amount of the red fragment and then deposit it at the center of the senile plaque. It is particularly the 1-42 amino acid piece of that protein which seems to be the bad toxic part (Figure 9). Now if we look at a senile plaque, we will find a variety of other molecules that are deposited there around the inflammatory reaction of the Aβ. So we really do have kind of a tombstone in a graveyard of brain damage occurring.

I'll just go through it once more. Under normal circumstances, we all make this protein, we all put it in

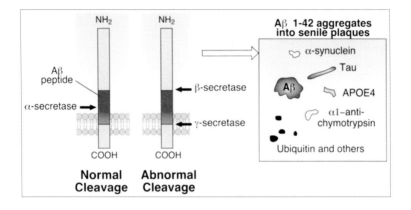

Figure 8

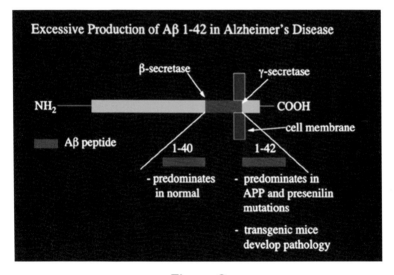

Figure 9

the membranes of our nerve cells and we all metabolize it and turn it over and α-secretase does that job. But in the abnormal circumstance, in the genetic conditions that have been mentioned, the cleavage of it occurs predominantly at the two ends of the red portion and the Aβ peptide gets deposited in the brain. It's particularly the 1-42 amino acid piece that causes the damage and the reason we think this is so important is that this fragment predominates in those genetic cases in which mutations occur in the amyloid precursor protein. The same thing can be produced in transgenic mice when gene defects are introduced into them.

These data suggest very strongly that in circumstances like mutations in the APP, where the 1-42 portion of the Aβ peptide predominates, it has a remarkable capacity to bind to itself. So, if one piece of this molecule forms, and it is like sticky glue, and attaches itself to another piece of itself, these form fibrils (Figure 10). Eventually these fibrils form clumps and the clumps form the plaques. It is the early part of this stage, when these fibrils are just beginning to come together, where therapy will be critical. It is at this time that they are so damaging to the nerve cells in the region.

Now I will move to where the science is taking us, specifically in terms of therapies that hopefully might change the course of these illnesses. I will introduce a general concept, not only in Alzheimer's disease but also in all of the other degenerative conditions that I referred to, where the common abnormality is that proteins get aggregated and clumped, that clump is toxic, and nerve cells die. If we look at Alzheimer's specifically, one could imagine that if these two enzymes are producing excessive

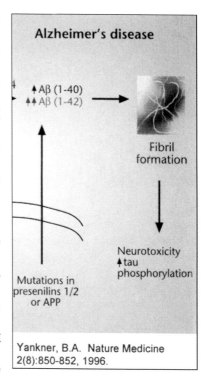

Alzheimer's disease

↟ Aβ (1-40)
↟↟ Aβ (1-42)

Fibril formation

Neurotoxicity
↟ tau phosphorylation

Mutations in presenilins 1/2 or APP

Yankner, B.A. Nature Medicine 2(8):850-852, 1996.

Figure 10

amounts of the Aβ, a good way to stop that would be to inhibit those enzymes; to develop a small molecule or drug that would, in fact, block the enzymes' actions and prevent them from forming the amyloid. That ought to work both in the rare instance of genetic or familial Alzheimer's as well as in the sporadic cases of Alzheimer's.

That effort is underway in probably a dozen or more pharmaceutical companies at the moment, who are trying to develop molecules that would inhibit the γ-secretase. Many inhibitors have been identified and they are extremely potent and effective in the animal models. They will prevent, in an animal with mutation, the deposition of amyloid. Several companies are now going forward with early phase clinical trials in humans. The reason this is so promising is that during the last 10-15 years, most of the new drugs that have come along and have really been powerful in changing the course of a disease have been enzyme inhibitors.

One can start with the angiotensin-converting

enzyme inhibitors, or the ACE inhibitors, which were discovered in the '80s. It is estimated that 10% of the population is on one of those for control of blood pressure. Then one has the statins, which have become so important in the management of hypercholesterolemia. They prevent the synthesis of cholesterol. Then protease inhibitors, which have been so successful in the treatment of AIDS, and tyrosine kinase inhibitors, for chronic myelogenous leukemia. The last is based upon the innovation of an oncogene that causes the leukemia to occur. So, the rationale behind going toward enzyme inhibitors as a successful treatment is based strongly and firmly in our recent experience.

The schematic diagram in Figure 11 (Page 26), prepared by my colleagues from the University of Washington in Seattle, offers a summary of our discussion and reminds us that most cases of Alzheimer's disease are not genetic. The rare cases that I referred to that are due to the mutations of APP genes PS 1 and PS 2

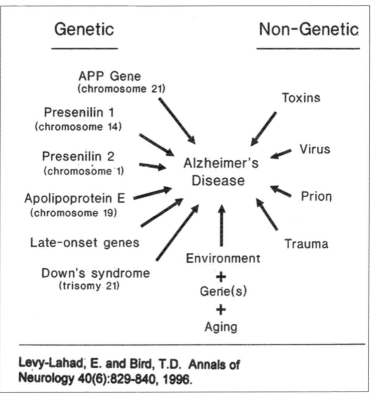

Genetic | Non-Genetic

APP Gene
(chromosome 21)

Presenilin 1
(chromosome 14)

Presenilin 2
(chromosome 1)

Apolipoprotein E
(chromosome 19)

Late-onset genes

Down's syndrome
(trisomy 21)

Toxins

Virus

Prion

Trauma

Alzheimer's
Disease

Environment
+
Gene(s)
+
Aging

Levy-Lahad, E. and Bird, T.D. Annals of
Neurology 40(6):829-840, 1996.

Figure 11

as a group only make up perhaps 3 to 5% of all cases of Alzheimer's. The association with apolipoprotein E does increase the risk for Alzheimer's. Very interestingly, Down's Syndrome, which was formerly referred to as mongolism, is associated with the duplication of DNA on the chromosome where amyloid is made, and every patient with Down's Syndrome who lives beyond age

40 develops Alzheimer's disease. This again confirms the hypothesis that excessive production of this material appears to be important in the causation of the disease.

There are, however, a variety of other things that impact this, some of which we know very little about and some of which we know something about. For example, it is well shown that head trauma increases the risk for later development of Alzheimer's disease and we know that educational level has some protective effect. There may well be toxins in the environment, although aluminum is not one of them, and the prion connection is not that prions cause Alzheimer's but that the mechanism of the new disease is similar, as we will see later. In thinking about this illness, one has to really put together the environment, genes, and of course, the most important risk which is growing old.

I return now to the protein aggregates (see Table 4 on next page) that I referred to, which are the basis for understanding the mechanisms of cell deaths and

Protein Aggregates in Neurodegenerative Diseases

Disease	Protein Deposits	Mutant Gene in Familial Disease
Prion disease	PrP amyloid plaques	PrP
Alzheimer's	$A\beta$ amyloid plaques	APP, PS1, PS2, ApoE, α2M
Parkinson's	α-synuclein in Lewy bodies	α-synuclein, parkin
Frontotemporal dementia	Fibrils	Tau
Huntington's	Huntingtin in nuclear aggregates	HD

Table 4

therapies. If we go to the prion disorders, which I will come back to, this is a problem with the prion protein (PrP). In the case of Parkinson's disease, by studying a very rare case of familial Parkinson's' disease, it was possible to identify a protein called α-synuclein which deposits in the brain in clumps as well. There is another form of Parkinson's disease, called juvenile Parkinson's disease, which occurs in childhood. It is associated with another mutation in a gene called Parkin.

Just before I leave the Alzheimer's story, I want to make one final point: how our cells work and how transmission of information occurs from the outside of

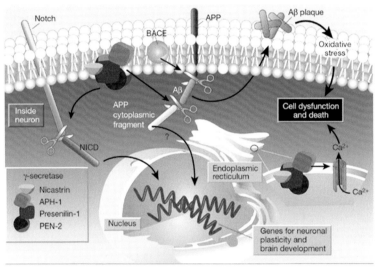

Figure 12

the cell to the inside, and then to the cytoplasm and to the nucleus (Figure 12) is a complex process. Let us look at the function of the secretase. They are represented in the diagram by two pairs of scissors which are cutting the Aβ protein to produce the material that we don't like. The reason they clip that is that the end piece of that protein probably has an important function, perhaps crossing over into the nucleus and telling genes in the nucleus to turn on or turn off. The important part of this diagram is that any one of these enzyme functions is more complex than a single pair of scissors cutting at one place. And, in the case of Alzheimer's, it appears that a clump of different enzyme proteins are involved in actually cutting the Aβ peptide.

The reason this is important is that the same clump of enzymes also cuts other pathways — in the diagram, the notch pathway — and it means that in finding a treatment that is specific for Alzheimer's disease, one has to find one that does not impact another pathway which is very important for development and cell connections. That is complicated but we must understand that selective γ-secretase inhibitors will have to prove not to be damaging to the cell.

Parkinson's Disease

Let's look at protein inclusions in the brain in general. Figure 13 (see Page 32) offers some pictures of a variety of diseases of which there will be more detail. One is the classic Lewy-body that is associated with Parkinson's disease, and then we have the infamous cytoplasmic occlusion of Huntington's disease. In the case of Huntington's disease, the protein Huntington is abnormally formed and it causes a central deposition within the nucleus in the parts of the brain affected by this condition and by some process that leads to cell death. In the case of α-synuclein in Parkinson's disease, the diagram shows deposition in the cytoplasm of the Lewy-body and some fibers in the brain that stain for that protein. Down below are plaques and tangles to which we have been referring. So, each of these conditions seems to be associated with these kinds of

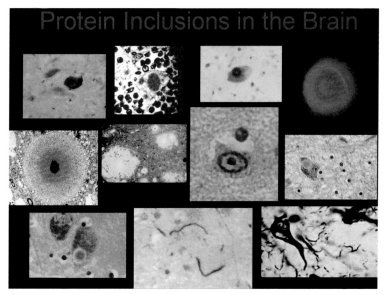

Figure 13

molecular changes.

Let's move a bit further now down the pathway of hope. Elucidating brain functions in health and disease might in fact lead to successful therapies. I will start with models of disease, which reminds me of an extraordinary talk about understanding how to use models of ALS and Huntington's disease to determine the mechanism by which cells die. This mechanism is referred to as programmed cell death. If you catch a cell and twinge it the wrong way, it automatically will kill itself to get out of the way and that series of cascades has been well worked out. Transgenic mice allow us to look at these diseases *in vivo* in an animal system where we can begin to test for things that would protect the animal or us from the illness.

There are a lot of studies now that are being done in coelacanths, which is a little worm about a millimeter in length. Its entire genome has been sequenced just like ours. It has 951 cells and 309 nerve cells. It has become a very important model since many of the genes that are identified in humans can actually be manipulated in the worm including point mutations (single gene abnormalities) that lead to prolonged life.

But I want to talk about the fruit fly with Parkinson's disease and show how these animal models can be so powerful in elucidating structures that will allow us to form new treatments. Now Parkinson's disease is much more common, as I mentioned. It is usually sporadic and only occasionally genetic and the genetics have helped us understand something about it. The onset is usually later in life although there are juvenile patterns of the disease and it is associated with slow movement called bradykinesia with postural instability, rigidity, and with the characteristic tremor that all of us have seen in a loved one, friend, or colleague. It is common; under age 50, perhaps 1 in 200 people, and over age 60, 1 in every 50-100.

The pathology of Parkinson's disease is shown in Figure 14, together with our friend the fruit fly. One can see that in the brain stem of the normal individual there is a pigmented nucleus called the substantia nigra which contains the cells that manufacture the dopamine, which is so important for the normal motor functions of the basal ganglia. In fact, L-Dopa replacement is the one treatment we have had for the last 30 years. In the patient with Parkinson's disease, the cells in that substantia nigra area die, the pigment is lost, and the projections from those cells into the basal ganglia are lost and dopamine deficiency occurs in the critical movement control centers in the basal ganglia.

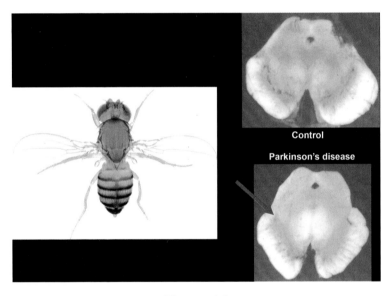

Figure 14

Fruit flies are interesting because they have dopamine cells, not a lot of them though, but they do not have the protein α-synuclein, the gene for which, if faulty, can cause Parkinson's disease. So what some investigators did at Harvard Medical School was they took a fruit fly which you can manipulate genetically quite easily and gave it the bad gene of Parkinson's disease.

The fruit fly now grew up with the gene that causes Parkinson's disease in us even though that gene wasn't normally present. As the right-hand-side diagram of Figure 15 shows, with those genes the nerve cells containing dopamine in humans die. When this protein is present in fruit flies, whether it is the normal protein or the mutated protein, the nerve cells that contain it die. So there is something very specific about this protein, α-synuclein, which when clumped in a cell containing dopamine causes it to die.

They even showed that these flies were not normal in terms of their movements and what they

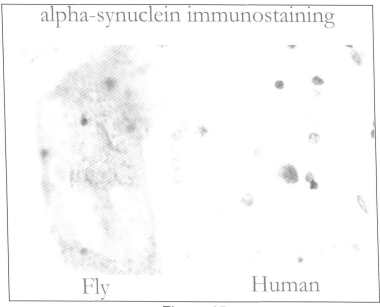

Figure 15

did was they took a bunch of flies and put them into a glass cylinder, tapped the bottom, and the flies climbed up to the top to get away from the noise. Then they calculated the percentage of fruit flies that could climb to the top (see chart in Figure 16). The normal fruit flies

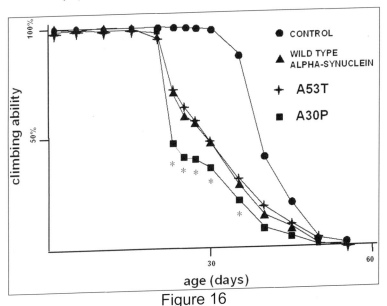

Figure 16

had no trouble at all so 100% of them did that. The fruit flies into which the gene, either the normal, so-called wild tab gene, or the mutated gene, was replaced began to show problems with movement at about 20-25 days and by the time they were 30-40 days old, were having great trouble with movement even though they lived an otherwise normal life. These fruit flies without the dopamine cells, which were killed when the gene for this protein was introduced, demonstrated motor problems very much like one would expect even in a higher species.

If one looks at the nerve cells that are dying (Figure 15), one can see the immunostaining in the fly is very similar in pattern to what occurs in humans. So these models of fruit flies that developed these kinds of symptoms can now be used for screening for drugs that might reverse that reaction. There are companies that have taken this model, not only for Parkinson's but for Huntington's and other diseases, and are using that to test drugs to see whether one can stop the deterioration that is associated with this effect. It becomes another model of disease and one can see in the electron microscope that the deposition is the same as in the humans.

Mad Cow and Other Prion Diseases

What we discussed so far has special relevance to Canada, and more specifically to Alberta. What we need to do is place the so-called Mad Cow crisis in perspective, in terms of both understanding what this illness is and in terms of the economics and how we assess risk in our society.

In 1996, when the full appreciation of the epidemic of Mad Cow disease was occurring in England, all of the imported cows that came from England were being killed in the United States. Newspapers ran stories of how strange an illness it seemed to be and we've all seen the horrible pictures of corpses of cows piled on top of each other. More than a million cows were destroyed, many of them infected, and despite that, there were only about 137 actual cases of variant Creutzfeldt-Jakob disease in the UK. With that huge

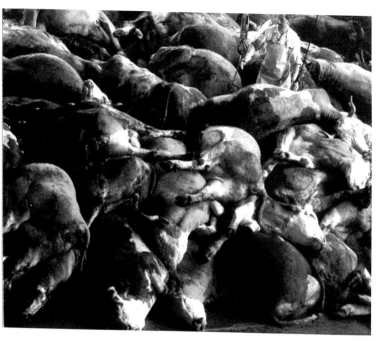

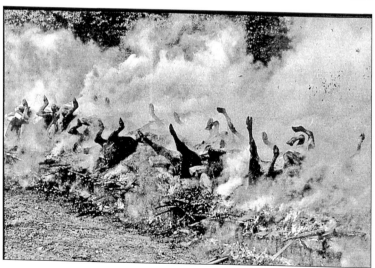

Mad Cows — End of the Line

number of cows infected, many of them were burned in order to try and render the possibility of transmission of the prion-protein from one cow to another to a minimum, that is, to prevent its spread in one way or another.

My father was a farmer and I grew up on a farm. I told him one day that I was studying Scrapey sheep and he said, "Oh I remember that!" and certainly many people in the eastern United States do remember that. I don't know whether Alberta has ever had Scrapey or not but it's a very common problem in sheep. It can cause their death and it's called Scrapey because they rub up against the posts in the corral and as a result of that, lose some of their wool.

Scrapey was not a worry to humans obviously. When it occurred the sheep might have been disposed of but there was no particular concern because they were not known to transmit whatever they had to any other species at all. It turned out that what they have in Scrapey is in fact a form of prion disease that is very similar to Mad Cow disease. More recently, this

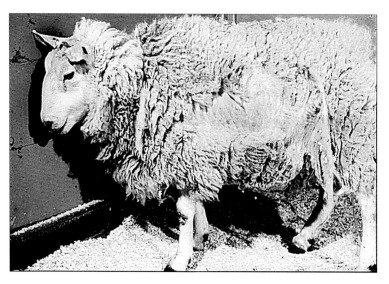

Figure 19: Scrapey sheep

concern has spread to the understanding that deer and elk can come down with what's called Chronic Wasting Disease (CWD), a fatal illness that causes weight loss.

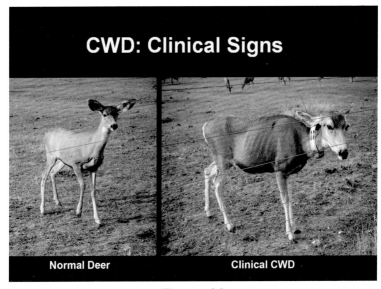

Figure 20

The distribution of this condition, or the areas of the U.S. and Canada where Chronic Wasting Disease has been found in captive populations, is shown in Figure 21 in the solid grey panels. The pink ovals are those sites, including one in Saskatchewan, where wild populations affected by this disease have been found.

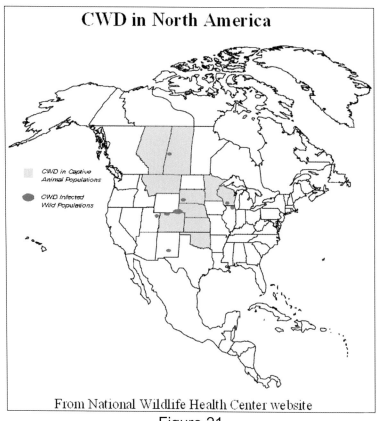

CWD in North America

CWD in Captive
Animal Populations

CWD Infected
Wild Populations

From National Wildlife Health Center website

Figure 21

This had raised a concern, a side issue, about whether eating such game meat could cause illness and, to date, there is no evidence at all that that is the case. There have been one or two cases of hunters in the U.S. who have died of Creutzfeldt-Jakob disease but this is within the infinites of that condition. It has never been shown that they actually got it from the tainted meat. Nevertheless, one of the other concerns we have is if, in fact, the prion-type illness can cross the species barrier.

Let me now go into the molecular biology of this group of disorders. They are truly bizarre and up until 10 years ago there was great skepticism about how this illness presented. It did, however, lead to one of our colleagues, Stan Prusner at the University of California San Francisco, being awarded the Nobel Prize for his heretical work, which began in the 1970s, around the theory about how prions caused this illness. Stan Prusner won the Nobel Prize in 1997 and he has become very involved in this set of issues worldwide as one of the leading experts. I have borrowed some of his material here.

What's strange about this prion set of disorders is it can be infectious, it can be inherited, or it can be spontaneous. Talking about being infectious, one might recall that 40 years ago in New Guinea a remarkable scientist called Karl Gadjusec noticed that in a tribe there the incidence of a shaking fatal illness was common and was particularly more common in women than in men. To make a long story short, it turned out that they obtained this infectious disease from cannibalism which was part of the rituals of the tribe and so the ingestion of human brain material that was infected with this disease led to the subsequent appearance of it in other members of the tribe.

He won the Nobel Prize for his hypothesis that this was due to an infectious agent which he showed could be transmitted to monkeys in his laboratory in Bethesda, Maryland. The brains from the patients who died in New Guinea could give the disease to chimpanzees or to other higher primates when injected into their brain. It's now known that there are no viruses involved and that this is an instance, whether it's infectious, inheritable, or spontaneous, where the infectious agent is actually a protein and furthermore, it's one of our own proteins which we all have. I'll now try to describe how it goes bad.

The image here shows this spongiform

Figure 22

encephalopathy that appears in the brain on modern scans and one can see, literally, holes punched in the brain from the loss of brain cells. So the mechanism of the disorder goes like this. In the normal circumstance, the prion protein, which we all have in our brain cells everywhere, has a shape (left-hand side diagram in Figure 23), of which the pink ribbons are called α-helices, which are structured in a particular way, and they have some blue terminal branches that come off them. For reasons that still remain mysterious, sometimes that protein in that three-dimensional structure changes to the shape shown on the right-hand side diagram, where a piece

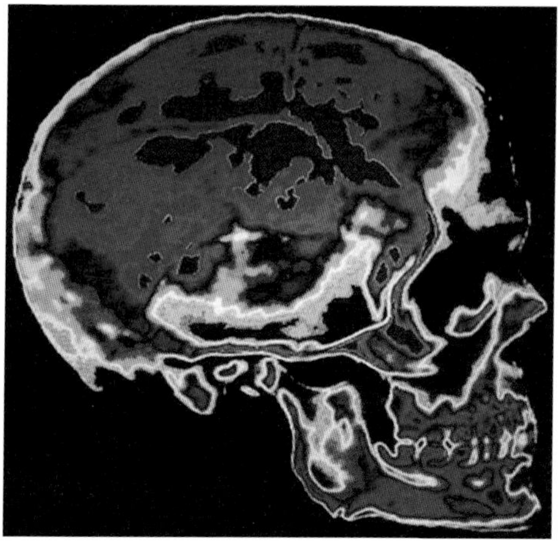

Conversion of α-helices into β-sheets in the prion protein is the fundamental event in prion diseases

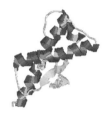 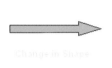 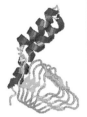

α-helices (corkscrew domains) in PrP^c are converted into β-sheets (flattened regions) resulting in the formation of PrP^{Sc}.

PrP^{Sc} which is rich in β-sheets accumulates in neurons and causes nervous system dysfunction

Figure 23

of the protein, not the α-helices in pink but the other part of it, become stacked together and accumulates in what is called a β-sheet. This transformation from the normal to this one here results in an infectious protein which then collects others like it, transforms some of the normal to it, and together they clump and form deposits in the brain which are the toxic materials that kill brain cells.

What turns out is that in this transformation or conversion from one to the other, there are a number of factors that can influence how easily that happens. They include other proteins which have been designated protein X that can occur in other mutations in which the PrP protein has a mutation, just like the ones in Alzheimer's, or when there are structural changes within the region that cause that transformation from one to the other to occur.

If we go back to our genetic model, what has been learned over two decades of genetic work with this disease in familial patients is that if you do a simple change in one base pair which can modify a single amino acid, one can end up with a host of possibilities here for genetic causes and mutations in this protein.

Each one of the points shown in blue in Figure 24 have now been associated with the development of the spongiform encephalopathy that is characteristic of this whole group of diseases. So genetic causes can occur but Creutzfeldt-Jakob is almost always sporadic and doesn't show any of these mutations that have been described here.

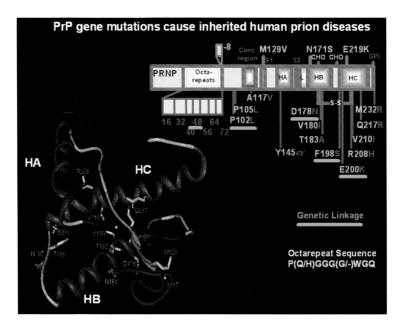

Figure 24

It is a curious disease as it can be infectious if you get it from a growth hormone which is purified from the pituitary. There was a batch of bad growth hormones in the 1980s that led to about 40 or 50 patients developing Creutzfeldt-Jakob. It occurred in patients with corneal transplants which had been inadvertently given to them from a patient who had the disease so it could be infectious, genetic, or sporadic.

Let me just make a few additional points about

changes in brain science that, hopefully, will lead to some new developments. I have already covered the last two of these but let me spend just a moment on brain plasticity. We recognize that the brain is not fixed, it changes during development, it changes during life, and is constantly modified in relation to experience. Plasticity in the brain occurs in learning and experience. Your brain, when you are leaving the room tonight, will be different from the brain you came in with. So there is a constant remodeling of the brain that occurs with everything that we do and most of this is based upon the plasticity of the synaptic connections between the brain cells, of which there are trillions.

It has been shown that synaptic plasticity actually can occur very rapidly; there could be a change in the shape of the connections between the synapses of the brain, there could be a change in their number, or in their density. We hope that we can learn about regeneration after injury to use these aspects of brain plasticity to treat spinal cord injury and so on.

Michelangelo and the Human Brain

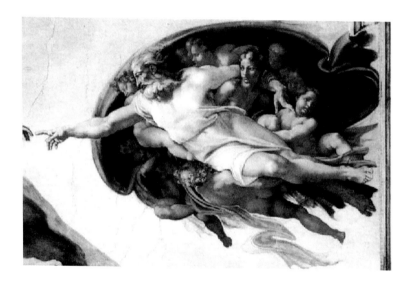

I want to take you on a little adventure here which came as a total surprise to me. You will recognize the image above, a part of the centerpiece of the Sistine Chapel that Michelangelo painted in 1510. In 1510, Michelangelo was a consummate expert in human anatomy, in understanding how things work. We know that he did dissections to help define the structures of muscles and the structure of the brain and so on. If one takes a close look at this figure of God creating Adam, those who do neuropathology will immediately recognize that this is the sagittal section of the human brain. The frontal lobes, the cerebellum, all are there. It also becomes obvious that God is the motor strip that carries down into the brain stem. One can also see portions of some cranial nerves, the basilar artery and the pituitary stock which I used to work on.

Now, is that a figment of my imagination or of Michelangelo's work? I was at the Sistine Chapel two years ago after its restoration and a lady beside us said, "Do you know that that's a sagittal section of the human brain?" I said, "No, I didn't know that." I had no idea who she was but she went on to fill me in on this. Upon my return, I did in fact discover some papers in recent literature. One was in the *Journal of the American Medical Association* which speculates that, in fact, Michelangelo did know enough about the brain to conceive of God as a figment of our imagination. I hope Michelangelo was not presenting this to suggest, as a central theory, that the brain is us.

Finally, I would point out that if one looks at the creation of Adam, that's a synapse. So, nearly 400 years before the word 'synapse' was termed, Michelangelo knew exactly what it was.

Stem Cells

The subject of stem cells is of immense research significance. Ground breaking stem cell research is well under way at the University of Calgary under the leadership of Dr. Sam Weiss. We share the hope that stem cells will lead to regeneration and repair. We know there are different kinds and we know that sometimes you can switch one into another kind, so let me give here just a quick course in stem cells.

The prospect here is that one can use stem cells directed and targeted for tissue regeneration in a selected area when damage occurs or when one wants to repair something. Cells capable of forming new tissue are identified in almost all organs; so there are cardiac stem cells, there are a lot of liver stem cells, skin reproduces itself regularly, and the intestine also does.

Stem cells that give rise to those specific cellular regions are well known. The argument in thinking about how this might impact on the future of medicine is that we recognize that as we grow older many of the conditions we face are associated with degeneration which makes up more and more of the healthcare burden for society and the hope is that one can find some way to alleviate the degenerative conditions that affect 128 million Americans.

What exactly is a stem cell? A stem cell is a cell that is capable of immortality by self-renewal. A stem cell divides into two daughter cells, one of which is a cell blanket which you can divide again, or into a second differentiated cell which is then capable of forming the tissue that that stem cell gives rise to, whether it is brain or muscle, bone, or bone marrow. This system is responsive to physiologic stimuli so that when you take a liter of blood out to give to the Red Cross, your bone marrow goes to work immediately, stem cells divide and the blood is re-formed to take the place of the blood lost. The differentiated cells, therefore, could become important for tissue repair or for developing therapies. The terminology here is important and the ethics and bioethics of it have to be understood around this terminology.

At the time of fertilization, the sperm and the egg produce the very earliest embryo (it is not called an embryo until it divides a certain number of times), but the first cells that are formed after the egg and sperm join are totipotential cells (Figure 26); they can become a whole human being. When they go further to what's called a blastocyst there are then a group of cells called the inner cell mass which can be taken out and which are shown to be pluripotent and capable of producing all the tissues of the body although they can not regenerate another human being. Those cells are called embryonic stem cells. When the fetus goes on to further development, you can take stem cells from that fetus, as has been done in the treatment of Parkinson's disease using the substantia nigra neurons. One can

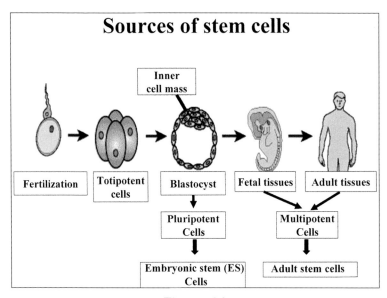

Sources of stem cells

Inner cell mass

Fertilization | Totipotent cells | Blastocyst | Fetal tissues | Adult tissues

Pluripotent Cells | Multipotent Cells

Embryonic stem (ES) Cells | Adult stem cells

Figure 26

also take particular bone marrow cells from adults and use them as we do so successfully in bone marrow transplants.

The issues that surround us in the U.S. are about the use of these embryos for medicine. The differences between therapeutic cloning and reproductive cloning has not always been, I think inappropriately, appreciated. Reproductive cloning is where you try to use this to produce an individual, which I'm sure we are all deeply opposed to. Whereas therapeutic cloning is where you take an embryo with the piece of skin or other tissue combined with an egg that is able to allow it to develop to the stage where one could take the embryonic stem cell and use it for therapeutic objective.

The world is very confused on this. Different countries have different rules as you know. In the U.S., at the moment we are only permitted to use a group of about 65 cell lines that were identified by the President two and a half years ago. Only about 15 of those are available and very recently at Harvard, one of our colleagues has developed some additional lines with private funding. The uses of stem cell technology is akin to using replacement parts to understand the mechanisms of development so that you can think about new ways to develop drugs and other approaches.

At this point, I would like to tell you about two things. One is the recent formation of the Harvard Stem Cell Institute that includes the Harvard Center for Neurodegeneration and Repair. I urge that you, in this community, think about that as a structure to take opportunities that your scientists here provide and go forward. The Harvard Stem Cell Institute has just been formed in the last few months with the idea of taking basic science to clinical treatments. It involves multiple schools at Harvard; the Faculty of Arts and Sciences, Harvard Medical School, and our teaching hospitals. It involves other schools at Harvard including the Business School, the Kennedy School, the Law School and very importantly, because the ethics of this are so important, the Divinity School.

University-wide faculty are involved too. Those of you who are scientists here will recognize Doug Melton and David Scadden. Doug is at the Faculty of Arts and Sciences and he is the one who has developed 17 new cell lines. He just announced those in the last couple of weeks. David Scadden is a clinician at the Massachusetts General Hospital and you will recognize a number of investigators such as Ole Issacson, who has done a lot of work in the nervous system, Chris Walsh, who has done a lot of work on brain development, and

Stu Orkin, who has done a lot of work on the stem cells in the bone marrow. You can find more information on the internet at www.isscr.org.

I want to conclude with the notion of why it is so important to do what you are talking about doing here today with the Calgary Brain Institute. Collaboration is critically important for advancing our science. Technology is increasingly interdisciplinary. It is the physicist, the chemist, the mathematician, the computer scientist who talks to the biologist, and, together, these are the specialists who will guide us to the future. It is expensive; we need to reduce redundancy, we need to enhance the likelihood of innovation and let me tell you about the experiment that we have now been undertaking for the past three years.

A very generous and anonymous donor in Boston contributed $37 million over a five-year period because he believed that if we had the seed funds to put together our community around the problems of neurodegeneration and tissue repair, he would be able to get us to work together in a way that might not otherwise happen.

He followed the model that we put together for our cancer center which does involve the entire Medical School and its hospitals. So we developed the five different cores: the Center for Translational Research, which includes a center to facilitate clinical trials, the Center for Brain Imaging, the Center for Molecular Pathology, a laboratory for drug discovery, and a Center for Bioinformatics.

The members of this group, which now totals more than 500 people, are scientists, principal investigators, all the teaching hospitals at Harvard who work in this area, and the basic science departments at the Medical School: biological chemistry, cell biology, genetics, neurobiology, pathology. The laboratories here are spread around the Medical School and its hospitals. It's a virtual set of activities but with cores that are available to anybody who wants to go to the imaging unit. We support MD and PhD students with this funding.

One of the very innovative parts of this is to take the step between basic science and the pharmaceutical industry, and so the Laboratory for Drug Discovery in Neurodegeneration is specifically screening in biological capacities that have to do with neurodegeneration for small molecules that might be promising for drugs. This was noted in *Science* a year ago — biotech thinking comes to academic medical centers where Ross Stein and Peter Lansbury who head this effort were noted for their efforts to bring into house management of science that will hopefully be the bridge to the pharmaceutical industry.

One of the things we are very proud of there is the Centre for Translational Neurology Research. We find more PhD students who actually want to come and work on these kinds of problems at the beginning. There are MD/PhD students who want to focus on neurodegeneration. So I would urge you here in Calgary, with the resources that are available and with the leadership that's in place, to think about how to create in this community the kind of interactive science that will lead to some of the important discoveries that are possible.

This field is so big and there are so many things to do, it is not all going to be done in one place. It will be done here, it will be done in Montreal, it will be done in Boston, it will be done in San Francisco.

Acknowledgments

Finally, to acknowledge some of the colleagues who lent me their slides: Fred Kolund, who works with Stan Krusner at UCSF, Susan Lindquist, who is head of the Whitehead Institute in Boston, Dennis Selkoe, who is with me as a Co-Chair of the Harvard Center for Neurodegeneration and Repair, Peter Lansbury, David Scadden, Doug Melton, and Mel Feeny, who is the young pathologist who developed the fruit fly report on Parkinson's disease.